HEARTBEATS

YOUR BODY, YOUR HEART

by Dr. Alvin & Virginia B. Silverstein

illustrated by Stella Ormai

J.B. Lippincott   New York

Heartbeats: Your Body, Your Heart

Designed by Ellen Weiss

Library of Congress Cataloging in Publication Data
Silverstein, Alvin.
    Heartbeats.

    Summary: Explains how the heart works, what happens
when it doesn't do its job properly, and the progress
made in the treatment of heart disease.
    1. Heart – Juvenile literature.   2. Heart – Diseases –
Juvenile literature.   [1. Heart.   2. Heart – Diseases]
I. Silverstein, Virginia B.   II. Ormai, Stella, ill.
III. Title.
QP111.6.S53 1983   612′.17   82-48465
ISBN 0-397-32037-X
ISBN 0-397-32038-8 (lib. bdg.)

1 2 3 4 5 6 7 8 9 10

First Edition

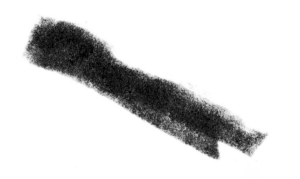

HEARTBEATS
YOUR BODY, YOUR HEART

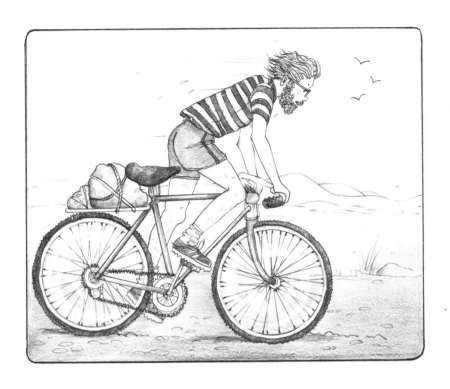

Recently a man named Jim Hayes rode his bicycle 3,000 miles across the country. Not many people could do something like that, but Jim Hayes was even more special. Five years before, he had had a heart transplant. His own heart could not work well enough to keep him healthy. He would have died if doctors had not given him a new heart.

Heart disease kills more Americans each year than anything else. Most of these people are middle-aged or old. So you may think that heart disease is just for old people. But young people can have bad hearts, too. Jim Hayes was only twenty-four when he had his heart transplant. Even babies can have heart disease.

Scientists have been studying heart disease for many years. They have been trying to find out more about what causes it, and have been searching for better ways to treat it. Scientists have not yet found a cure for heart disease. But what they have learned is helping to save lives. Even though heart disease is still the biggest killer in the United States, it is not killing as many people as it used to. Each year fewer people die from heart disease than the year before.

What is the heart? Why is it so important? What does it do in the body?

You probably think you know what the heart looks like. But you probably are wrong. The heart does not look very much like the shapes people draw on Valentine's Day. And it certainly isn't flat, like a paper valentine. A real, live heart is shaped something like an ice-cream cone, with a pointed bottom and a rounded top, like two scoops of ice cream. It is hollow and can fill up with blood. A grown-up's heart is about the size of a large orange. It weighs a little less than a pound.

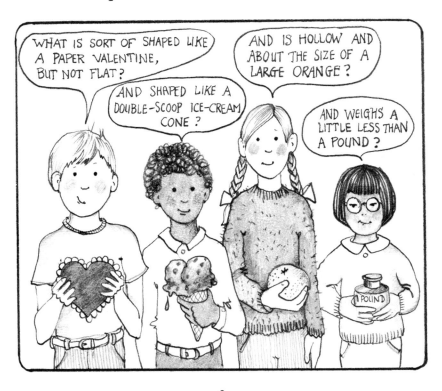

When you pledge allegiance to the flag, you place your hand over the left side of your chest. Do you know why? That is supposed to be where the heart is. Actually, the heart is in the middle of the chest. It fits in snugly between the two lungs. But the heart is tipped over, so that there is a little more of it on the left side than on the right. The pointed tip at the bottom of the heart touches the front wall of the chest. Every time the heart beats, it goes *thump*

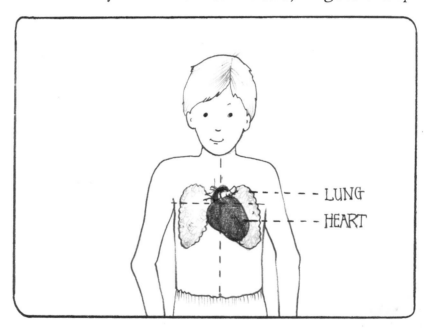

LUNG

HEART

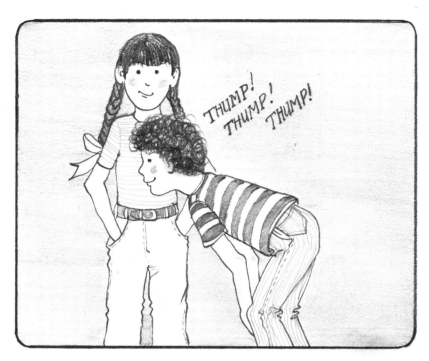

against the chest wall. You can feel the thumps if you press there with your hand. You can hear them with your ear.

The heart is a pump. Its walls are made of thick muscle. They can squeeze (contract) to send blood rushing out. The blood does not spill all over the place when it leaves the heart. It flows smoothly in tubes called blood vessels. First the blood flows into tubes called arteries. The arteries that leave the heart are thick tubes. The biggest one, called the aorta, is an inch wide. But the arteries soon branch again and again, to form many smaller tubes. These blood vessels carry blood to all parts of the body. The farther from the heart, the more blood vessels there are, and the smaller they are. The tiniest blood vessels, called capillaries, are so small you would need a microscope to see them. Capillaries join to form larger blood vessels. These tubes carry blood back toward the heart. The bigger ones are called veins. The closer to the heart, the fewer the veins there are, and the larger they are. The largest veins empty blood into the heart.

So the blood vessels of the body carry blood in a circle: moving away from the heart in arteries, traveling to various parts of the body in capillaries, and going back to the heart in veins. Scientists call the heart and blood vessels the circulatory system. They say that blood circulates in the body. And the heart is the important pump that makes this happen.

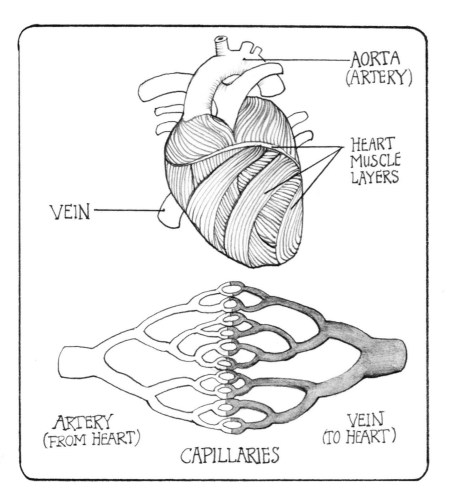

AORTA
(ARTERY)

HEART
MUSCLE
LAYERS

VEIN

ARTERY
(FROM HEART)

VEIN
(TO HEART)

CAPILLARIES

If you could look inside your heart, you would see that a wall of muscle divides it down the middle, into a left half and a right half. The muscular wall is called

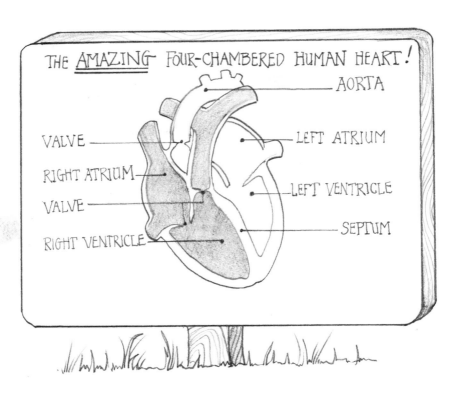

THE <u>AMAZING</u> FOUR-CHAMBERED HUMAN HEART!

- AORTA
VALVE -
- LEFT ATRIUM
RIGHT ATRIUM -
VALVE -
- LEFT VENTRICLE
- SEPTUM
RIGHT VENTRICLE -

a septum. Another septum separates the rounded top part of the heart from the cone-shaped bottom part. So there are actually four chambers (spaces) inside the heart. Each top chamber is called an atrium (plural: atria). The bottom ones are called ventricles. Blood can flow from the atria down into the ventricles, because there are openings in the walls that separate them. But blood cannot flow back and forth between the left and right halves of the heart. The septum that separates them is solid.

The atria are the receiving chambers of the heart. Blood flows into them from the veins. The ventricles are the pumps, and their walls are thick and strong. When they contract, they send blood rushing out through the arteries.

The circulatory system is actually made up of *two* circles. The left ventricle of the heart sends blood out through the big artery called the aorta. From there it flows into the branching arteries that carry it to various parts of the body. The veins that carry blood back from the body parts empty the blood into the right atrium of the heart. The blood then flows down into the right ventricle, which pumps it into a different circle of blood vessels. This circle goes from the right ventricle to the lungs and back to the heart, into the left atrium. From there the blood flows into the left ventricle. Then, in the next heartbeat, this blood is pumped out into the body again by the left ventri-

BLOOD FLOW

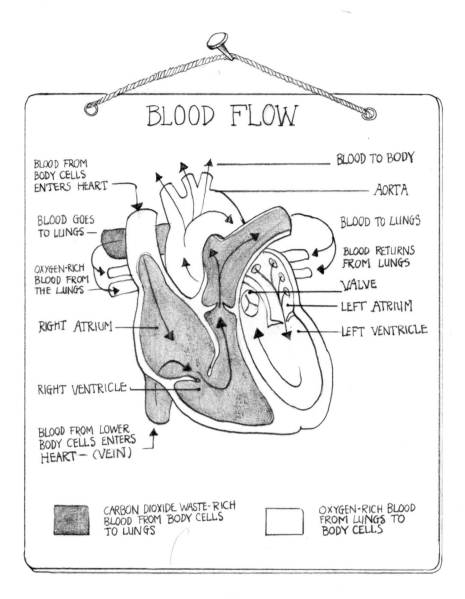

BLOOD FROM BODY CELLS ENTERS HEART

BLOOD GOES TO LUNGS —

OXYGEN-RICH BLOOD FROM THE LUNGS

RIGHT ATRIUM

RIGHT VENTRICLE

BLOOD FROM LOWER BODY CELLS ENTERS HEART — (VEIN)

BLOOD TO BODY

AORTA

BLOOD TO LUNGS

BLOOD RETURNS FROM LUNGS

VALVE

LEFT ATRIUM

LEFT VENTRICLE

CARBON DIOXIDE WASTE-RICH BLOOD FROM BODY CELLS TO LUNGS

OXYGEN-RICH BLOOD FROM LUNGS TO BODY CELLS

cle. The two circles of blood vessels are separate, but the heart is in the middle of each of them.

Why does the heart pump blood in two separate circles? The answer involves two important gases, oxygen (O_2) and carbon dioxide (CO_2).

All the cells of the body need energy to do their work. They get energy by combining sugars or other food materials with oxygen. This chemical reaction is something like burning. The chemical reaction in a burning fire gives off heat and light. The chemical reaction inside body cells gives off heat and other forms of energy. This energy provides the power we need to talk and move and think.

When a fire burns, carbon dioxide is formed. When a body cell combines sugar with oxygen to get energy, carbon dioxide is formed here, too. But too much carbon dioxide could poison a cell.

So all the body cells need some way to get oxygen. They also need some way to get rid of carbon dioxide. The blood does both these things. It brings oxygen to the body cells and takes away their carbon dioxide. These gases pass easily back and forth through the thin walls of the tiny capillaries.

Oxygen gets into the body when we breathe. Air contains oxygen. When you breathe in, air flows into your nose, down your windpipe, and into your lungs. Inside the lungs there are many tiny air sacs called alveoli. Each one is so small that you would need a microscope to see it. The walls of these little air sacs

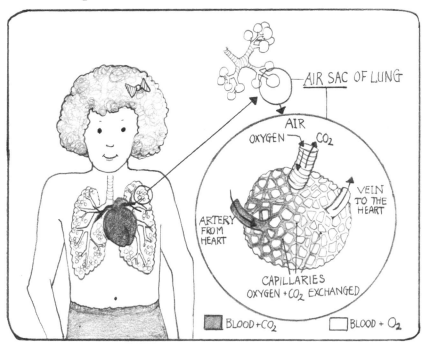

AIR SAC OF LUNG

AIR

OXYGEN CO_2

ARTERY FROM HEART

VEIN TO THE HEART

CAPILLARIES
OXYGEN + CO_2 EXCHANGED

BLOOD + CO_2 BLOOD + O_2

are very thin. They are wrapped in a network of tiny capillaries. Blood from the heart flows through these capillaries and collects the oxygen. The oxygen-rich blood is returned to the heart and pumped out to the body.

As the blood flows through the capillaries in the body, carrying its supply of oxygen, it also collects carbon dioxide. The blood that empties into the right atrium is dark colored. It has picked up carbon dioxide from the body cells. It has left most of its oxygen with the cells. This is the blood that the heart pumps into the lungs. We can think of the dark, carbon dioxide-rich blood as used blood.

In the lungs, carbon dioxide passes out of the capillaries into the tiny air sacs. When you breathe out, you get rid of this carbon dioxide. Oxygen from the air sacs passes into the blood capillaries, and the circle begins again. Even though it is the same blood that carried the carbon dioxide wastes, when it has unloaded them and taken on a new cargo of oxygen, we can think of it as fresh blood—it is as good as new.

Both oxygen and carbon dioxide are carried in the blood mainly by the red blood cells. These tiny cells look something like doughnuts without the holes in the middle. There are enormous numbers of red blood cells. You have about 250 *million* of them in each drop of your blood! An adult has about 6 quarts (5 liters) of blood altogether, containing about 25 trillion (25,000,000,000,000) red blood cells. These tiny cells are like little ferry boats. They float along in the blood, carrying their cargoes of oxygen or carbon dioxide.

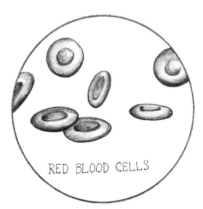

RED BLOOD CELLS

The oxygen-rich blood from the lungs is bright red. It empties into the left atrium. Then the left ventricle pumps it out into the arteries that lead to the body.

The heart never rests. Your heart started beating about eight months before you were born. It will beat over 2½ billion times in your lifetime. In all those years it will never take a day off—not even a minute off. Your body needs the flow of fresh blood that the heart keeps pumping.

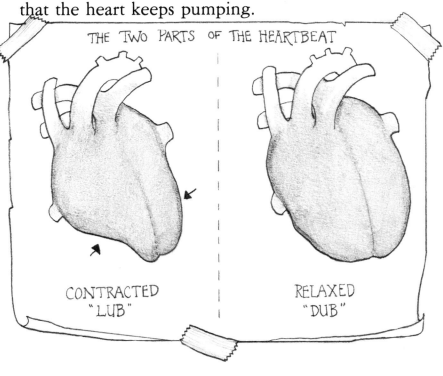

THE TWO PARTS OF THE HEARTBEAT

CONTRACTED "LUB"

RELAXED "DUB"

What is a heartbeat? It has two parts. First the heart muscle contracts. The contraction starts with the atria, which push blood down into the ventricles. Then the walls of the ventricles squeeze together and force blood out into the arteries. The contraction is the first part of the heartbeat. After that, the heart muscle relaxes. The heart gets larger again, and blood can flow in from the veins.

Why doesn't blood flow back in from the arteries, the same way it went out? It can't, because the heart has some little trapdoors to stop it. These trapdoors are called valves. There is a valve at the bottom of the aorta, and another one in the large artery—called the pulmonary artery—that leads to the lungs. Trapdoor valves also guard the openings from the atria into the ventricles. So there is always one-way traffic in the heart. The valves keep blood from flowing backward.

If you listen to a person's chest with a stethoscope, you can hear the sounds of the heartbeat clearly. Each beat has two sounds, like *lub-dub.* The *lub* is a

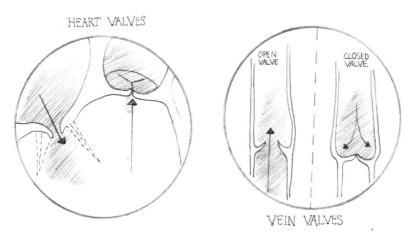

HEART VALVES

OPEN VALVE

CLOSED VALVE

VEIN VALVES

long, booming sound. The *dub* is a short, snapping sound. The *lub* is the sound of the ventricles contracting and the valves from the atria closing. When the ventricles start to relax, the valves to the arteries snap shut. That is the *dub* sound.

Usually the heartbeat is very regular, like the ticking of a clock. In adults, a normal heart beats an average of about 70 times a minute (a little faster than a clock ticks). Children usually have a faster heartbeat, about 90 times a minute. Women's hearts usually beat faster than men's. People who have trained for running or other sports have slower

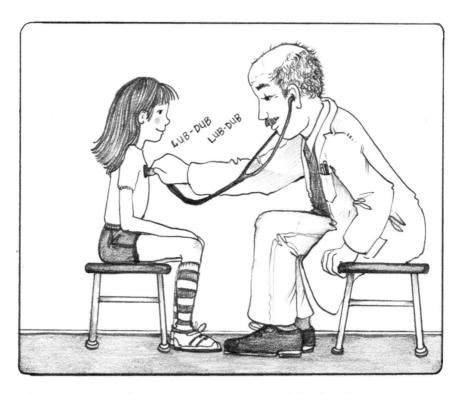

heartbeats than the average. Their hearts are strengthened by the exercise, so they can pump more blood in each beat. Athletes' hearts may need to beat only 50 times a minute or even less during rest. (They speed up during exercise, but not as much as the average person's heart does.)

Heart muscle can contract on its own. One part of

the heart muscle, called the pacemaker, acts as a built-in timer. It sends out tiny bursts of electricity—not enough to cause a shock, but enough to start the muscle contracting. The pacemaker sets the rate of the heartbeat and keeps all the parts of the heart working to the same rhythm.

Messages from the nerves can speed up or slow down the heart's pacemaker. That way the heart can speed up and pump blood faster when you are active and your body cells need more oxygen and food materials.

The body makes chemical messengers called hormones. These can also change the rate of the heartbeat. A hormone called adrenaline makes the heart speed up. It is produced when you are frightened or excited. It is your body's way of preparing you in case you may need to fight or run away. Do you ever feel as if your heart is pounding when you are frightened? That is adrenaline making your heart beat faster.

The heart is such a hard worker that it uses a lot

of oxygen and food materials itself. It has its own blood supply. Coronary arteries bring fresh blood to the heart. Coronary veins drain the used blood away.

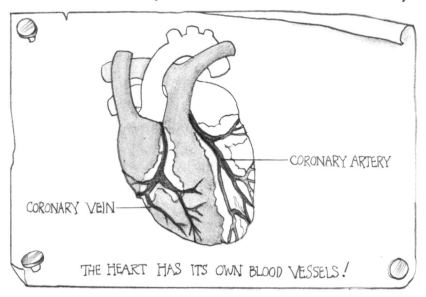

CORONARY ARTERY

CORONARY VEIN

THE HEART HAS ITS OWN BLOOD VESSELS!

It might seem silly for the heart to have its own blood vessels. After all, the heart fills up with blood, again and again, with each heartbeat. But the blood that the heart pumps does not get inside the heart muscle. It does not get to the heart muscle cells that do the work.

It is amazing that most hearts keep on working so

well, for so long. (You wouldn't expect a car's engine to keep on running for seventy years.) But there are many things that can go wrong with the heart, or with the blood vessels connected to it.

Some babies are born with hearts that did not form properly. For example, there might be a hole in the septum that separates the right ventricle from the left one. That kind of heart defect causes two problems. First of all, the heart does not pump as well as it should. When the ventricles contract, part of the blood goes rushing out through the arteries the way it should. But part of the blood just swishes around, back and forth through the hole between the ventricles. That is bad, but the second problem is even worse.

In a normal heart the right ventricle fills up with used blood from the body cells. This blood carries a lot of carbon dioxide and very little oxygen. The left ventricle fills up with fresh blood from the lungs. This blood has a lot of oxygen and very little carbon dioxide. If there is a hole in the septum, the two kinds of blood mix. The mixed blood does not have as much oxygen as the fresh blood, and it has more carbon dioxide. The used blood doesn't all make the circle to the lungs. So the blood the heart sends out by the aorta to the body cells does not have as much oxygen as it should, and it has too much carbon dioxide. This blood cannot give the body cells enough of the oxygen that they need. So they cannot work as well as they should.

Another kind of heart defect can cause the same problems. Before a baby is born, it lives in a watery fluid inside its mother's body. It does not breathe. (If it did, it would breathe water, not air!) So it does not get oxygen through its lungs. Oxygen comes from the mother's blood. The mother's blood and the baby's blood do not mix. They flow in their own separate circulatory systems. But in the placenta, where the baby is connected to its mother's body, some of the blood vessels are close together. Gases like oxygen and carbon dioxide can pass through the thin walls of the capillaries. Oxygen crosses over

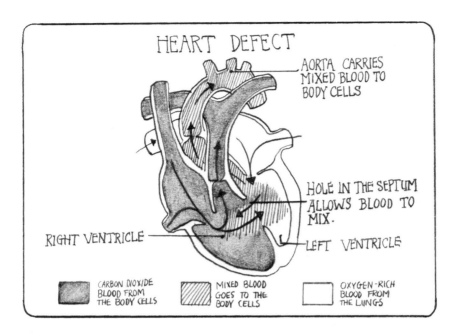

HEART DEFECT

AORTA CARRIES MIXED BLOOD TO BODY CELLS

HOLE IN THE SEPTUM ALLOWS BLOOD TO MIX.

RIGHT VENTRICLE

LEFT VENTRICLE

CARBON DIOXIDE BLOOD FROM THE BODY CELLS

MIXED BLOOD GOES TO THE BODY CELLS

OXYGEN-RICH BLOOD FROM THE LUNGS

from the mother's blood to the baby's. Carbon dioxide goes the other way.

Before birth, there is a little blood vessel connecting a baby's aorta with its pulmonary artery—the one that leads from its heart to its lungs. Much of the blood pumped out of the right ventricle goes right around and into the aorta, avoiding the detour through the lungs, the left atrium, and the left ventricle. (Remember, the baby's blood does not need to go to the lungs to get oxygen.) After birth, the baby breathes air, and it needs a circulatory system with two separate circles. The connection between the aorta and the pulmonary artery closes. But sometimes this does not happen. Then the oxygen-rich blood from the left ventricle can mix with the oxygen-poor blood from the right ventricle.

Babies with heart defects that allow the two flows of blood to mix are called blue babies. The blood that flows through their bodies is darker than it should be. That makes their skin look blue. These babies do not grow as well as they should. They feel weak and tired. Their hearts may get very large from trying to pump more blood to the body cells that need more oxygen than they are getting. After years of working too hard, their hearts may break down and stop pumping.

Years ago, children born with heart defects usually died very young. But today doctors have many tools to use to diagnose heart problems—to find out what is wrong. And they have ways to fix heart defects so that the children can grow up and live a normal life.

Listening through a stethoscope can tell a heart doctor whether the heart is pumping properly. If there is a hole in the septum, for example, and the blood is mixing, there are extra swishing noises. Faulty heart valves that do not close all the way when the heart pumps also make noises the doctor can hear. These extra noises are called heart murmurs.

Heart murmurs can be a sign of a heart defect. But many people with normal hearts have heart murmurs too. Usually doctors can tell which kinds of heart murmurs are signs of problems. But if they are not sure, there are many other tests they can use.

X rays can show doctors what a person's heart looks like. The newest X-ray machines can give a picture of any part of the heart. Or they can even show a "movie" of the heart beating, which doctors can watch on a TV screen.

The echocardiograph is another kind of machine for "seeing" into the heart. It uses ultrasound. This is sound so high-pitched that humans cannot hear it.

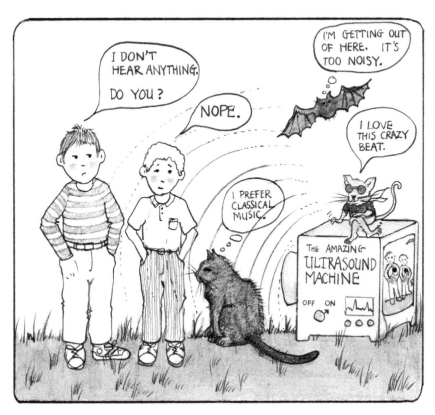

(Cats, mice, and bats can hear ultrasound.) The echocardiograph bounces ultrasound waves off the heart, and the "echoes" form a picture.

The electrocardiograph is a machine that records electricity from the heart. Did you know that your heart produces electricity? It is not enough to give you a shock if you touch your chest. But electrodes pasted to the chest can pick up the heart's electricity. They give the doctor a record of every heartbeat. This record may be traced as a squiggly line glowing on a screen. Or a pen may draw the electrocardiogram on graph paper. (The tracings are known as

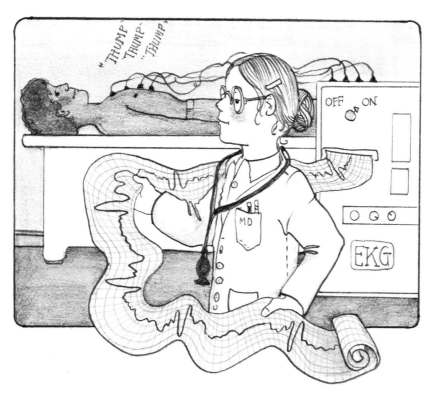

EKGs.) A doctor can look at the tracing and tell if the heart's pacemaker and valves are working properly, and if the heart muscle is pumping as it should.

Heart doctors can fix many kinds of heart defects. Sometimes they have to operate on the heart, but sometimes that is not necessary. For example, scientists have found a drug that makes the connection between the aorta and the pulmonary artery close up. A hole in the septum can be fixed with a pair of tiny patches that are injected into a vein and literally pushed up to the heart, through the blood vessels, on a long wire. When the two parts of the patch are in place, they open up like tiny umbrellas and snap together. The wire can then be pulled back out of the vein.

Heart-lung machines have made it possible for doctors to operate on the heart. During the operation, the person's blood flows through a machine that puts in oxygen and takes out carbon dioxide. That way, the doctor can stop the person's heart and work on it while it is not moving. (Imagine how hard it

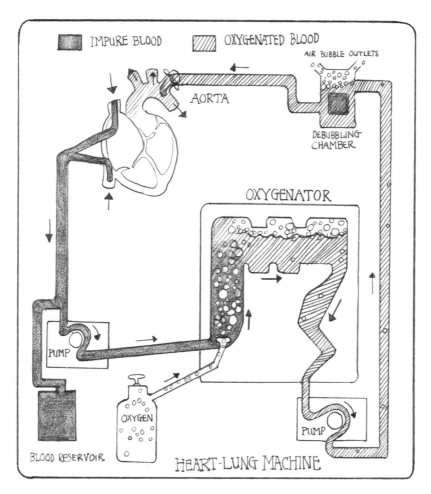

IMPURE BLOOD | OXYGENATED BLOOD

AIR BUBBLE OUTLETS

AORTA

DEBUBBLING CHAMBER

OXYGENATOR

PUMP

OXYGEN

PUMP

BLOOD RESERVOIR

HEART-LUNG MACHINE

would be to try to fix up a heart while it was beating!) The doctors can sew up holes and open blocked arteries. They can even move arteries around if they did not grow in the right place. If there is something wrong with the heart valves, doctors can put in new ones. Sometimes they use valves from pig hearts. Or they may put in artificial valves. There are also artificial pacemakers. Doctors can put one in to set the heartbeat rate if the heart's own timer is not working properly.

What causes heart defects? Sometimes they are the result of something that happened to the mother while her baby's heart was forming. If the mother gets rubella (German measles), her baby may be born with a heart defect. Drugs like Thalidomide can also damage a baby's heart if its mother takes them while the heart is forming.

Doctors do not always know what caused a heart defect in a newborn baby. But they do know what causes many heart problems in children and teenagers. That is rheumatic fever.

Did you ever go to the school nurse to have a throat culture when you had a sore throat? It's not much fun to have the nurse poking a swab in your

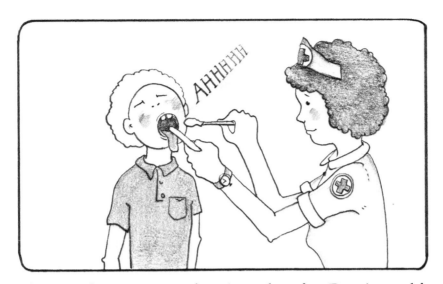

throat when you are hurting already. But it could save you a lot more pain later. Some sore throats are "strep throats." They are caused by a germ called *Streptococcus.* Many sore throats quickly get better by themselves. Strep throats seem to get better, too. But sometimes the strep germs stay hiding in the body. The throat doesn't hurt anymore, but after a couple of weeks the child may have a fever and sore joints. This is rheumatic fever. Knees, elbows, and other joints ache painfully because they are swollen. The strep germs are there, and the body is fighting them.

Strep germs may also attack the valves in the heart. The valves get swollen, and afterward they may be scarred. They may not work properly any longer.

Rheumatic fever does not have to happen anymore. Antibiotics, taken when the child has a strep throat, will kill the strep germs and keep them from attacking the joints and the heart. You can't tell whether a sore throat is a strep throat just by the way it feels. But a throat culture is a quick and easy test

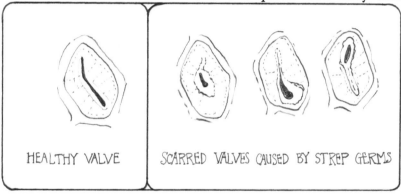

HEALTHY VALVE   SCARRED VALVES CAUSED BY STREP GERMS

to tell the difference. Many children whose hearts are damaged by rheumatic fever could have stayed healthy if they had had throat cultures done. But they didn't bother because they thought it was "just a sore throat."

Heart defects and rheumatic fever can cause heart disease in children. But most people who suffer from heart disease are grown-ups. Doctors think that the kind of heart disease most people get develops very slowly. It takes years. And it does not start in the heart. It starts in the arteries.

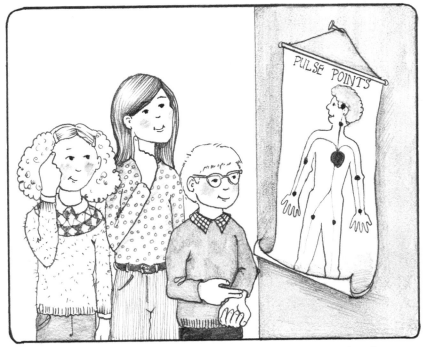

The arteries that carry blood through the body are tubes with thick, muscular walls. After each beat of the heart, the artery walls contract too. They help to pump the blood along. You can feel the beating of your arteries in places where they pass close to the surface. This beat is called the pulse. Usually people take a pulse at the wrist. But you can also feel a pulse in your neck, at your temples, and in other places, too.

In a young child, the insides of the arteries are smooth and slippery. Blood flows through them easily. But then little lumps of fatty material may stick to places inside the arteries. These little fatty patches are called plaques. As the years go by, the fatty plaques may grow bigger. Calcium salts may be added to them. Then they become hard, like bits of rock.

When this happens, the arteries cannot work as well as they should. They are getting clogged up with plaques, so the hole for blood to flow through is getting narrower and narrower. Their walls are getting stiff and hard, so they cannot pump the blood along as well as they used to. When the arteries are

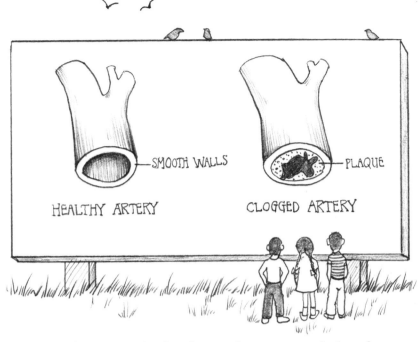

HEALTHY ARTERY   CLOGGED ARTERY

hard and clogged, the heart has to work harder to pump blood through them. The heart may grow larger, trying to pump enough blood through the stiff arteries. The heart may get so large that it is like a stretched-out rubber band that can't snap back the way it should.

When the coronary arteries get clogged up with fatty deposits, not enough blood can flow to the heart muscle. The heart cells do not get all the oxygen they need. Then the person may feel a sharp pain called angina. The pain is a signal. The starved heart cells are calling for help. Hard work, walking fast, or excitement may make the pain worse. That happens because the heart is trying to work harder and needs even more oxygen than usual.

Hardening of the arteries does not usually start to cause heart problems until middle or old age. But the plaques begin to build up much earlier, even in the teen years.

When the heart cannot work as well as it should, it does not move enough blood through the body. Fluid from the blood leaks out through the walls of the tiny capillaries, and it collects in the tissues of the body. The person's face and hands and feet may get puffy and swollen. Fluid stays in the lungs and makes it harder to breathe. The kidneys do not get enough blood flowing through them. Normally, the job of the kidneys is to clean waste products and poisons out of the blood. But if the heart does not send enough blood through the kidneys, they cannot clean the blood. Some poisons stay in the blood and are carried to the body cells. They make the person feel sick. This kind of heart disease is called congestive heart failure. People talk about heart disease as the number one killer, but it is a crippler, too. It causes many years of misery for millions of people.

As the arteries get narrower and harder, the space inside them for blood to flow through gets smaller and smaller. Eventually an artery may close up completely. Or, even more likely, a small blood clot may plug it up.

Blood clots can save lives. If you cut yourself, blood flows out at first. But then it stops. A dark red lump forms in the cut. This is a blood clot. After a while it turns into a hard scab. The scab protects the cut while new skin is growing. When the cut is healed, the scab falls off.

If you could look at a blood clot under a microscope, you would see that it is made up of a net of tiny fibers. The threadlike fibers are sticky, and blood

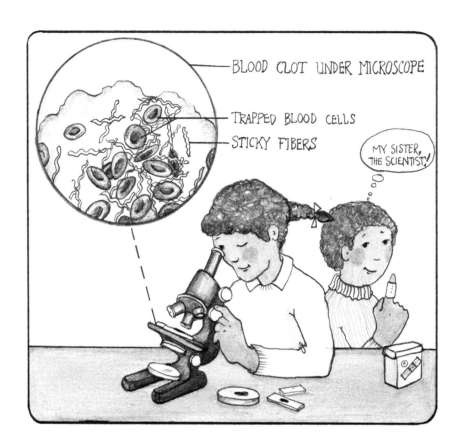

BLOOD CLOT UNDER MICROSCOPE

TRAPPED BLOOD CELLS

STICKY FIBERS

cells get caught in them. The clot forms a patch to keep any more blood from leaking out. Chemicals in the blood react to form clots. Some people are born without some of the special blood-clotting chemicals. Their blood does not clot properly. They can bleed to death from just a small cut, unless they take special medicines to make their blood clot.

Blood clots are not supposed to happen *inside* a blood vessel. They should form when blood vessels are torn or cut. Delicate little structures called blood platelets catch on the rough edges of the cut and tear open. They spill out the chemicals that help to make a clot form.

But plaques are rough. Sometimes they tear the delicate blood platelets inside a blood vessel. And then a clot may form inside. That kind of blood clot may kill!

There are chemicals in the blood that break up blood clots. Usually these chemicals take care of any stray clots before they can do any harm. But if plaques have made the arteries very narrow, a clot may stick in a narrow spot and plug it up. No blood can flow past the plug.

What happens then? That depends on where the plug formed. Sometimes nothing happens. Many parts of the body get blood from several different arteries. If one gets plugged up, the cells will still get the oxygen and food materials they need from the other arteries. But some parts of the body have only one blood supply. If that artery is blocked, the cells will be starved. If the plug is not cleared away quickly, cells will start to die. This is called infarction.

If a blood clot plugs up an artery leading to the brain, the person may have a stroke. In a stroke, blood cannot get to part of the brain. Without the oxygen and food materials the blood carries, brain cells will be starved and die. The person may lose the ability to speak, or to move an arm or even one whole side of the body. If enough brain cells die, the person will die.

If a plug forms in one of the coronary arteries that supply the heart, part of the heart muscle will die. That is what happens in a heart attack. If only a small part of the heart muscle is hurt, the heart can keep on working. But it may not work as well as it used to. Then, if the person has another heart attack, there may not be enough healthy heart muscle left to keep on beating.

What causes heart disease? How can it be prevented? How can people who have it be helped? Doctors don't have all the answers yet. But they are making progress on all these problems.

Have you heard people talking about "cholesterol"? That is a fatty substance found in foods like meat and eggs. Cholesterol is the main fatty substance in the plaques that clog up arteries. Studies have shown that people with a lot of cholesterol in

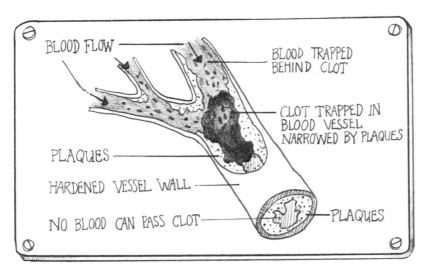

their blood are more likely to get heart attacks. So for a while doctors thought that eating foods with cholesterol was one of the main causes of heart disease. But the story is not really so simple.

Nerve cells and other body cells need cholesterol. We get some in the foods we eat, but the body can make cholesterol, too. In fact, if you eat less cholesterol, your body may make more of it. Scientists have found that the cholesterol in the blood does not stay there by itself. It becomes attached to fats called HDLs (high-density lipoproteins) and LDLs (low-density lipoproteins). The HDLs are the "good guys" in the cholesterol story. They help cholesterol to get into the cells where it is needed. The LDLs are the "bad guys." They help cholesterol form plaques inside arteries. So now doctors don't just measure cholesterol in a person's blood. They look for HDLs and LDLs, too. And scientists have been trying to find ways to make the body make more HDLs and fewer LDLs.

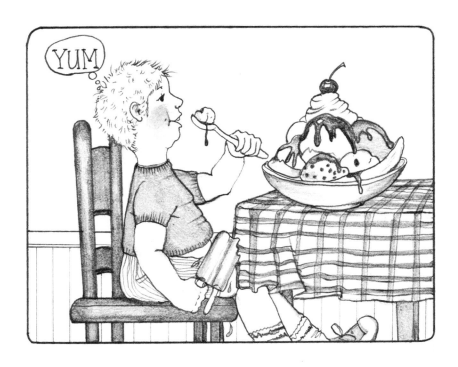

Eating too much fat is one way to increase your risk of getting heart disease. Eating too much sugar is bad, too. (The body has ways of changing extra sugar into fat.) In fact, eating too much anything is bad, if you eat so much that you get overweight. When a person is gaining weight, the body makes more LDLs, and fatty plaques form inside the arteries. Overweight is also bad because the heart has to work harder to pump blood through all that extra fatty tissue.

People who are overweight are also more likely to have high blood pressure. When the blood pressure inside the arteries is high, the heart has to work harder to pump blood through them.

Exercising regularly is good for the heart. Exercise helps to burn up food materials and keep a person from getting fat. Scientists have found that exercising makes the HDLs (the "good fats") go up and the LDLs (the "bad fats") go down. And exercise makes the coronary arteries grow extra branches. Then they can bring more blood to the heart. If one artery gets blocked, the heart cells won't die, because blood can get to them through different branches.

Smoking is bad for the heart. Heavy smokers are twice as likely to have heart attacks as people who don't smoke. The nicotine in cigarettes speeds up the heart and makes it need more oxygen. It also narrows the arteries, so that the heart has to pump harder.

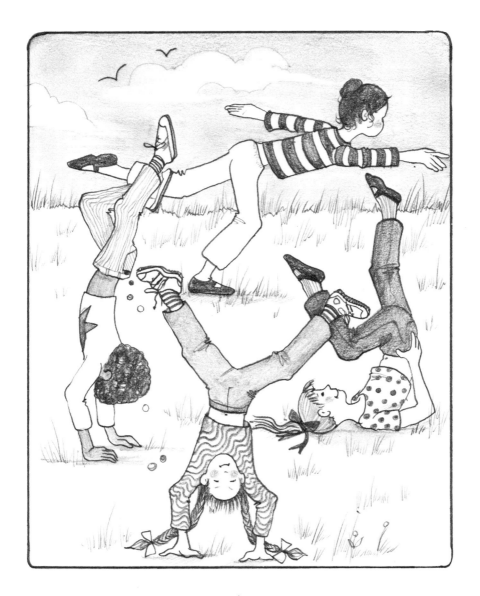

And it makes blood more likely to clot. Cigarette smoke also contains carbon monoxide. That is the same gas that is in car exhausts. Carbon monoxide goes into red blood cells. If they are carrying carbon monoxide, they can't carry oxygen. And yet a smoker's heart needs even more oxygen than usual. So smoking may cause attacks of angina, the pain that means heart cells are starving.

Many scientists think that stress is an important cause of heart disease. People who try to work too much—and worry about it—are more likely to have heart attacks. That is one kind of stress. Another kind is caused by too much noise. Loud noises, worries, and other upsetting things cause the body to make adrenaline. Remember, that is a chemical that can speed up the heart. The blood pressure also goes up. Too much stress, too often, can wear out the heart and blood vessels.

The foods we eat, exercising, smoking, and stress— these are all parts of the way we live that can help or hurt the heart. And yet they do not have the same effects on everybody. The kind of body you have can make a difference, too. Doctors are now finding that heart disease can be hereditary. Some people's bodies cannot handle fats as well as others. Even when they follow a normal diet, they have too many LDLs, and plaques form in their arteries. In some cases this can even happen in children. Fortunately, very few children die of heart attacks. But people with the hereditary kind of heart disease may have heart attacks when they are young adults.

Doctors use many different kinds of drugs to treat heart disease. There are drugs that help keep the blood from clotting inside the arteries. Other drugs help to clear the fatty plaques out of arteries. When the heart's pacemaker is not working as well as it should, there are drugs that can help to keep it beating steadily.

Better treatments for high blood pressure are helping to bring down the number of deaths from heart disease. A test for high blood pressure is quick and easy. Doctors and nurses test all their patients for it.

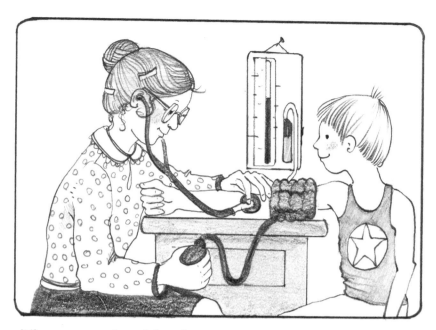

There are also blood pressure testing machines in many shopping centers. There are even some that people can use on themselves at home. Often people do not know they have high blood pressure until a test shows it. But once they know, there are drugs and other treatments that can bring the blood pressure down to normal. One thing that helps is to eat less salt. Doctors think that most people eat too much salt, and that can cause high blood pressure.

When heart attacks do happen, quick treatment can save lives. Calling the doctor right away is important. But even that may not be quick enough. If the heart stops pumping, the brain cells will be starved. The victim may die in just a few minutes. Many people are learning how to do CPR (cardiopulmonary resuscitation), which is a way to keep a heart attack victim alive until the doctor comes. CPR does not need any special machines or equipment. A person who has been trained in this first-aid method presses on the victim's chest to keep the heart pumping and breathes into the victim's mouth to send air into the lungs.

If a person is having chest pains and is not sure if it is really a heart attack, doctors have good tests to use. An electrocardiograph picks up the tiny bursts of electricity from the heart and traces out heartbeat waves. Doctors looking at the EKG tracings can tell if the heart is damaged and where the trouble is. They can also test the blood for certain chemicals that tell if a person has had a heart attack.

In former times when people had heart attacks, all any doctor could do was to keep them very quiet and hope the heart would heal itself. But now doctors have ways to keep the heart muscle from getting damaged. When a clot is blocking a coronary artery, there are drugs that can clear the clot away. If these drugs are given fast enough, the blood starts to flow through the artery again. And then the starving heart cells do not die. Other drugs, given after a heart attack, help to strengthen the heart and increase its blood supply. These drugs are helping to save people who would soon have had second heart attacks.

When a heart is too badly damaged to be fixed, surgeons may try a heart transplant. They take out the damaged heart and put in a new one from someone who has died in an accident. The first heart transplant was done in 1967. There were a lot of problems that had to be solved. For example, the body has defenses against "foreign invaders" like germs. Somebody else's heart has "foreign" chemicals that set off the body's defenses. So the person may "reject" a new heart because the body's defenses attack it. Tests have been worked out to match up the person and the new heart as closely as possible. Doctors can also use drugs and other methods to stop the body's defenses from attacking the transplant. So there are now many people alive who have transplanted hearts.

But heart transplants could never help large numbers of people—not the millions who suffer from heart disease. For each person saved by a heart transplant, someone else has to die. So scientists have also been working on artificial heart parts and even a complete artificial heart.

Thousands of people have artificial heart valves. Thousands have artificial pacemakers, which send out electrical signals to set a steady heartbeat. A left ventricular assist pump can help out for a while after a heart operation. It gives the heart a chance to rest and heal. The most exciting advance of all is the use of a completely artificial heart. Seattle dentist Barney Clark was the first man to receive a permanent artificial heart. This was the Jarvik-7. But there are problems. The Jarvik-7 must be connected by hoses to an outside power source. The patient cannot move more than six feet from the machine. Soon other heart patients will receive artificial hearts with a built-in power source. These artificial hearts will work just as well as a real heart, for years and years.

Meanwhile, other researchers are working on new and better ways to treat and prevent heart disease. They hope that someday it will be a very rare disease, not the number-one killer it is today.

Here are some words you might want to use in talking about heart disease. Words in SMALL CAPITALS are defined in their own entries.

---

adrenaline—a HORMONE that speeds up the heartbeat rate.

alveolus (*pl.*, alveoli)—a tiny air sac in the lungs.

angina—a sharp pain that is felt when heart cells are not getting enough oxygen.

aorta—the largest ARTERY in the body. Blood empties into it from the left VENTRICLE of the heart.

arteriosclerosis—HARDENING OF THE ARTERIES.

artery—a BLOOD VESSEL that carries blood away from the heart.

atrium (*pl.*, atria)—an upper chamber of the heart that receives blood from VEINS and empties it into a VENTRICLE.

blood vessel—a tubelike structure that carries blood.

capillary—a tiny BLOOD VESSEL with very thin walls, through which gases are exchanged with the cells.

carbon dioxide—a gas given off by the cells in the production of energy.

cholesterol—a fatlike substance found in the PLAQUE that clogs an ARTERY. (It is also an important part of nerve cells.)

congestive heart failure—an illness in which the heart cannot pump enough blood, and, as a result, body tissues fill with fluid, fluid in the lungs makes it hard to breathe, and the kidneys cannot remove all the poisons from the blood.

coronary artery—an ARTERY that carries oxygen-rich blood to the heart muscle.

coronary vein—a VEIN that drains oxygen-poor blood from the heart muscle.

CPR (cardiopulmonary resuscitation)—a first-aid method to keep HEART ATTACK victims alive until the doctor comes, by pressing rhythmically on the victim's chest and breathing into his or her mouth.

EKG (electrocardiogram)—a tracing of the waves of electrical activity from the heart.

electrocardiograph—a machine that traces the heart's electrical activity.

hardening of the arteries—the formation of fatty PLAQUEs in the ARTERY walls, which are hardened by deposits of calcium salts.

HDLs (high-density lipoproteins)—fats in the blood that help carry CHOLESTEROL into the cells where it is needed.

heart attack—sudden damage to the heart muscle that results when its blood supply is cut off.

heart murmur—sounds that can be heard through a STETHOSCOPE when the blood is not flowing smoothly through the heart.

heart transplant—the replacement of a badly damaged heart by a healthy heart from someone who has died in an accident.

hemophilia—a hereditary disease in which blood-clotting chemicals are lacking and the blood does not clot properly.

high blood pressure—higher than normal pressure in the arteries, so that the heart has to work harder to pump blood through them.

hormones—chemical messengers, carried in the blood, that help to control body activities.

hypertension—HIGH BLOOD PRESSURE.

infarction—death of cells when their blood supply has been cut off.

LDLs (low-density lipoproteins)—fats in the blood that help to carry CHOLESTEROL into fatty deposits (PLAQUEs) in the ARTERY walls.

nicotine—a drug in cigarettes that speeds up the heart, narrows the arteries, and makes blood clot faster.

oxygen—a gas found in air that combines with food materials in the body cells to produce energy.

pacemaker—a specialized part of the heart muscle that sets the regular heartbeat rhythm.

plaque—a fatty deposit in an ARTERY wall.

platelets—delicate structures in blood that help to form blood clots.

pulmonary artery—an ARTERY that carries blood from the heart to the lungs. Unlike the other arteries, the pulmonary artery carries oxygen-poor blood.

pulmonary vein—a VEIN that carries blood from the lungs to the heart. Unlike the other veins, the pulmonary vein carries oxygen-rich blood.

rheumatic fever—a disease that may follow a STREP THROAT and causes damage to the heart VALVEs.

septum (*pl.*, **septa**)—a muscular wall separating the chambers of the heart.

sphygmomanometer—an instrument used to measure blood pressure. See HIGH BLOOD PRESSURE.

stethoscope—an instrument used to listen to the heartbeat.

strep throat—a throat infection caused by the *Streptococcus* bacterium.

valve—a trapdoor-like flap that permits the flow of blood in a BLOOD VESSEL to go in one direction only.

vein—a BLOOD VESSEL that carries blood toward the heart.

ventricle—a lower chamber of the heart, which receives blood from an ATRIUM and pumps it out into an ARTERY.

adrenaline, 19, 46, 53
alveolus (*pl.*, alveoli), 12,
    53; see also: lungs, air
    sacs of
angina, 36, 46, 53
anticlotting drugs, 47, 50
aorta, 6, 7, 8, 9, 16, 23,
    24, 53
arteries, 6, 7, 33, 35, 53
arteries, hardening of,
    34–37, 54
arteriosclerosis, 53; see
    also: arteries, hardening
    of
artificial heart, 51, 52
artificial heart valves, 51
artificial pacemakers, 51
atrium (*pl.*, atria), 8, 9,
    16, 53

blood, 6, 13
blood, amount in body, 14
blood clot, 37–40, *38*, *41*
blood pressure testing
    machines, 48
blood vessels, 5, 6, 53
blue babies, 24
brain, 40, 49

capillaries, 6, *7*, 12, 13,
    36, 53
carbon dioxide, *10*, 11,
    13, 14, 21, 22, 28, 54
carbon monoxide, 46
cholesterol, 41, 42, 54
circulatory system, 6, 9
Clark, Barney, 51
congestive heart failure,
    36–37, 54
coronary arteries, 20, *20*,
    35, 40, 50, 54
coronary veins, 20, *20*, 54
CPR (cardiopulmonary
    resuscitation), 49, 54

echocardiograph, 25, 26
EKG (electrocardiogram),
    27, 28, 49, 54
electrocardiograph, 26, *27*,
    49, 54
energy, 11
exercise, 18, 44

German measles, 30

hardening of the arteries,
    34–37, 54

Hayes, Jim, 1, 2
HDLs (high-density
   lipoproteins), 42, 44, 55
heart, 7, 8, *10*
heart, artificial, 51, 52
heart, blood flow in, 9,
   10 11
heart, blood supply of, 20
heart, position of, 4
heart, shape of, 3
heart, size of, 3
heart, structure of, 7–9
heart attack, 40, 49, 55
heart defects, 21–25, *23*
heart defects, causes of, 30
heart defects, repair of,
   28–30
heart disease, causes of,
   41–47
heart disease, treatment of,
   47–52
heart-lung machines, 28,
   29
heart murmurs, 25, 55
heart muscle, *7*
heart sounds, *15*, 16–17
heart transplant, 1, 50, 51,
   55
heart valves, *8*, 16, *17*,

25, 30, 32, *32*, 57
heart valves, artificial, 51
heart valves, scarred, *32*
heartbeat, 4, 9, 15, *15*,
   16, 17, 18, 19
heartbeat rate, 17–18, 19
hemophilia, 55
heredity and heart disease,
   47
high blood pressure, 44,
   47, 48, 55
hormones, 19, 55
hypertension, 56; see also:
   high blood pressure

infarction, 40, 55

Jarvik-7, 52

kidneys, 36, 37

LDLs (low-density
   lipoproteins), 43, 44,
   47, 56
left atrium, 8, 9, *10*, 14
left ventricle, 8, 9, *10*,
   14–15
left ventricular assist pump,
   51

lungs, 4, 9, *10*, 13, 14
lungs, air sacs of, *12*,
    12–13; see also: alveolus

nicotine, 44, 56
noise, 46

overweight, 43, 44
oxygen, *10*, 11, 12, 13,
    14, 20, 21, 22, 24, 28,
    36, 46, 56

pacemaker, 19, 28, 47, 56
pacemaker, artificial, 51
placenta, 22
plaques, 34, 36, 39, *41*,
    42, 43, 47, 56
platelets, 39, 56
pulmonary artery, 16, 23,
    24, 56
pulmonary vein, 56
pulse, *33*, 34

red blood cells, 14
rejection of transplants, 51
rheumatic fever, 30–32, 57
right atrium, *8*, 9, *10*, 13
right ventricle, 9, *9*, *10*

rubella (German measles),
    30

salt, 48
septum, 8, *8*, 21, *23*, 25,
    28, 57
smoking, 44, 46
sphygmomanometer, 48,
    57
stethoscope, 25, 57
strep throat, 31, 32, 57
Streptococcus, 31
stress, 46
stroke, 40
sugar, 43

Thalidomide, 30
throat culture, 30, 32

ultrasound, 25

valve, *8*, 16, *17*, 25, 30,
    32, *32*, 57
veins, 6, 57
ventricle, 8, 16, 57

X rays, 25